CBD Oil: Learn How CBD Oil Can Naturally Treat Diseases And Improve Health

By

Cami Baker

Introduction

I want to thank you and congratulate you for downloading the book, *"CBD Oil: Learn How CBD Oil Can Naturally Treat Diseases And Improve Health"*.

This book has actionable information on how to make the most use of CBD oil.

The legalization of medical marijuana by many states in the recent past has brought about renewed interest into research about the many ways that marijuana can be of use. The primary focus of this research has been on CBD, the medicinally beneficial component of marijuana.

This research has unearthed a countless number of benefits that come with using CBD, among them reversing type II diabetes, fighting epilepsy, chronic pain, psoriasis, Parkinson's, and many others. Therefore, if you are struggling with these health problems or many others, you may be surprised that CBD oil might be the one thing that has been lacking in your treatments.

And this book will show you everything you need to know about CBD oil including what it really is, what makes it effective, the benefits that come with using CBD oil, where to get CBD oil, how to use it and much, much more!

Let's begin.

Thanks again for downloading this book. I hope you enjoy it!

© **Copyright 2018 - All rights reserved.**

This document is geared towards providing exact and reliable information in regards to the topic and issue covered. The publication is sold with the idea that the publisher is not required to render accounting, officially permitted, or otherwise, qualified services. If advice is necessary, legal or professional, a practiced individual in the profession should be ordered.

- From a Declaration of Principles which was accepted and approved equally by a Committee of the American Bar Association and a Committee of Publishers and Associations.

In no way is it legal to reproduce, duplicate, or transmit any part of this document in either electronic means or in printed format. Recording of this publication is strictly prohibited and any storage of this document is not allowed unless with written permission from the publisher. All rights reserved.

The information provided herein is stated to be truthful and consistent, in that any liability, in terms of inattention or otherwise, by any usage or abuse of any policies, processes, or directions contained within is the solitary and utter responsibility of the recipient reader. Under no circumstances will any legal responsibility or blame be held against the publisher for any reparation, damages, or monetary loss due to the information herein, either directly or indirectly.

Respective authors own all copyrights not held by the publisher.

The information herein is offered for informational purposes solely, and is universal as so. The presentation of the information is without contract or any type of guarantee assurance.

The trademarks that are used are without any consent, and the publication of the trademark is without permission or backing by the trademark owner. All trademarks and brands within this book are for clarifying purposes only and are the owned by the owners themselves, not affiliated with this document.

Table of Contents

Introduction

CBD Oil for Beginners

What Is CBD Oil?

CBD and the Endocannabinoid System

The Amazing Benefits of CBD Oil

Where to Find CBD Oil

How To Use CBD Oil

Possible Risks And Side Effects Involved

Conclusion

Before we get to a point of discussing the many benefits that you can get by using CBD oil, let's understand what it is first so that we are on the same page as we move forward.

CBD Oil for Beginners

What Is CBD Oil?

CBD, sometimes known as **cannabidiol,** is one of more than 80 other active cannabinoid compounds that occur naturally and are found in the cannabis plants.

Cannabis is an annual herbaceous flowering plant and CBD oil is typically extracted from the resin glands of the flowers and the buds of the plant.

Marijuana and hemp are examples of types of cannabis and therefore, cannabis does not necessarily have to mean marijuana. In fact, cannabis is the general umbrella term and the scientific genus name under which all types of hemp and marijuana lie.

Even though CBD oil is extracted from marijuana and hemp plants, it is not the substance that makes you feel 'high'. This means that you have nothing to worry about when using it to cure whatever ailment. The main psychoactive cannabinoid that produces the 'high' feeling of euphoria and relaxation is THC (tetrahydrocannabinol) by binding to the CB1 and CB2 receptors in the brain, which in turn makes the brain to have a high feeling.

The reason why CBD does not give you a high is because its interaction with these brain receptors is 100 times weaker than THC. In short, when CBD binds to the receptors, it does not in any way stimulate the ECS (endocannabinoid system) to release dopamine in the brain, which creates the high. CBD will therefore give you the same health benefits that marijuana does without altering your brain.

CBD oil is usually extracted from the cannabis plants that have low amounts of THC but have high contents of CBD such as hemp. The oil is extracted from the plant in three ways. It can be extracted by using carrier oil such as olive oil, using ethanol (high grain alcohol) or by using the CO_2 method whereby CO_2 is blown at high pressure through the plant at a cool temperature to extract a very pure form of CBD.

Next, we will be discussing about how CBD affects the endocannabinoid system.

CBD and the Endocannabinoid System

The discovery of the endocannabinoid system and how cannabinoids affect it was hailed as the most important medical discovery in the history of medicine since the sterile surgical method was invented.

The **endocannabinoid system** is an endogenous biological system that developed in the body of all vertebrae over 600 million years ago. This system plays a key role in maintaining of the neurophysiological processes such as regulation of body temperature, fertility, appetite, motor skills, sleeping cycle, emotions, pain, synaptic plasticity, development of the neuromuscular system, neuronal development etc; all of which amount to homeostasis.

Homeostasis is a physiological process that involves the whole body (all cells and tissue) to maintain the body balance, a general state of calm, serenity and wellness. This is a necessity if the body is to stay alive. Homeostasis also slows down aging and prevents various diseases from developing.

The endocannabinoid system is made up of **endocannabinoids** ('endo' means inside), endocannabinoid receptors such as (GPR55, CB1, CB2 and TRPV1) and enzymes whose function is to decompose and synthesize proteins and endocannabinoids in the entire nervous system. The endocannabinoid system can therefore be termed as a form of chemical-physical communication system that maintains homeostasis.

Endocannabinoids are fat-like molecules that bind to the same cannabinoid receptors just as **phytocannabinoids** (plant-based cannabinoids) do. CBD and THC are examples of phytocannabinoids.

Every organ in your body, including the skin and the digestive tract, all have cannabinoid receptors. Basically, these receptors exist in nearly every tissue and cell in your body. This is why CBD is believed to have an impact on every aspect of human health and behavior; from the sub-cellular level to the body in its entirety.

The plant based cannabinoids (phytocannabinoids) mimic these endocannabinoids. They help the body to recover from crises and return to a normal state when the body's own endocannabinoids fail to help the body recover on their own.

Experts have discovered that the endocannabinoid system can also respond to and recognize exogenous cannabinoids (cannabinoids from external sources), and especially cannabidiol. The [National Institutes of Health](#) have reason to believe that if you were to manipulate the endocannabinoid system by introducing external cannabinoids like CBD, then you would end up treating a huge number of medical ailments.

CBD essentially interacts with your endocannabinoid system, which is made up of millions of cannabinoid receptors that are spread across the entire body although most of them are found in the central nervous system and the brain. CBD interacts with these receptors to help ease pain, anxiety, insomnia and inflammation while also improving cardiovascular and neurological functions.

With the interaction between CBD and the endocannabinoid system, you can bet that there is likely to be some effects, which manifest in the form of health benefits. We will be discussing that in the next chapter.

The Amazing Benefits of CBD Oil

1. **Fights Anxiety and Depression**

For patients who suffer from obsessive compulsive disorder, panic disorder, post-traumatic stress disorder and social anxiety disorder, CBD has proven to be effective in combating such problems. In fact, further studies also show that CBD can drastically reduce the stage fright and anxiety caused by public speaking. Researchers found that patients who were treated with CBD recorded a significant reduction in discomfort, cognitive impairment, anxiety and they had a significant decrease in alertness in anticipation of their speech. Cannabidiol was also found to have an antidepressant-like kind of effect in rodents.

Sometimes depression develops because of Vitamin B12 deficiency. However, using CBD oil can reduce the level of depression by improving the signaling of both the glutamate cortical and serotonergic agents (which when in low quantities result into depression). The antidepressant effect of CBD on the human body is usually continuous and fast, over time; an effect that is similar to that of Tofranil (Imipramine).

2. **Relief From Chronic Pain**

Among the many amazing benefits that come with the use of CBD, relief from chronic pain tops the list for many patients. There is reason to believe that CBD oil and other non-psychoactive constituents of cannabis could represent a novel category of therapeutic agents for the management of chronic pain. Chronic pain is any pain that lasts for more than 12 weeks and can be as a result of an injury, or pain associated with diseases such as cancer.

In one study published in the *Journal of Experimental Medicine*, CBD was used on rodents and the neuropathic and chronic inflammatory pain they were suffering from reduced significantly. This was achieved even without causing analgesic tolerance. This means that the rodents were not likely to build tolerance to CBD and therefore wouldn't need to constantly raise the dosage as is the case with most pain killers.

More interestingly, the use of cannabidiol combined with THC produced promising results when used to treat chronic pain associated with rheumatoid arthritis, cancer, multiple sclerosis and fibromyalgia. This was according to a 2007 meta-analysis study conducted in Canada. Sativex was the name given to the combination of THC and CBD sublingual spray. Further studies also show that there are also other opioids, which can also be combined with CBD to help relieve pain.

3. **CBD As An Anti-Cancer Mechanism**

The role of CBD in the treatment of cancer still needs more studies. However, available research looks promising. Research shows that not only CBD alone but also other phytochemicals found in cannabis are capable of having an anti-tumor effect and could therefore be used to improve the usual medication.

This scientific report demonstrates how CBD possesses pro-apoptotic and anti-proliferative effects that together inhibit the invasion and adhesion as well as the migration of cancer cells.

In a 2011 study, scientists shed some rays of light on a cellular mechanism such that CBD would induce the death of cancer cells in breast tissues. They discovered that CBD generated a '*concentration-dependent cell death*' of both estrogen receptor-negative and estrogen receptor-positive breast cancer cells.

A 2006 study published in the *Journal of Pharmacology and Experimental Therapeutics* discusses how CBD selectively and potently inhibits the growth of different breast tumor cell lines displaying considerably less degree of potency on the healthy cells.

Treating cancer patients with CBD oil has been shown to strengthen the LAKs (lymphokine activated killer cells) thus killing the cancer cells more. Furthermore, cannabidiol also blocks the signaling of CPR55 thus decreasing cancer cell proliferation and bone reabsorption.

Studies suggest that CBD can also act as an anti-tumor agent to decrease human glioma invasion and cell growth. Elsewhere, CBD has shown to increase tumor cell death in both colon cancer and leukemia cases.

4. **CBD Prevents Nausea And Boosts Appetite**

If you've ever suffered from such irritating digestive disorders, then you know the negative impact they can have on your life. It is also well known that persons who consume cannabis tend to experience increased appetite.

Did you know that nausea has a lot to do with your mind? The uncomfortable feeling you get on your throat and stomach, sometimes accompanied by vomiting is usually as a result of an **imbalance** in your gastric movements by either chemotherapy, bacteria or virus.

But according to findings from the National Cancer Institute, cannabidiol binds to the cannabinoid receptors in your mind and body and this increases appetite rapidly. A separate study showed how effective CBD was as it helped relieve rodents from nausea and vomiting.

Interestingly, scientists have also discovered that when CBD is used in low quantities, it helps to curb the nausea and vomiting that is caused by toxic drugs.

When taken in high quantities however, it was shown to either have no effect whatsoever or it increased levels of nausea. This study was done on animal models thus more clinical studies proving the effectiveness of CBD are still needed in humans.

5. **CBD Treats Insomnia**

If you suffer from insomnia or struggle to get an undisturbed and restful sleep throughout the night, then you need to get your hands on the cannabinoid oil. There are thought to be many causes for restlessness and lack of sleep at night, but the greatest causes are anxiety and stress; which we've earlier seen can also be combated by using CBD oil.

Taking some before bedtime has been scientifically proven to improve the quality of sleep. CBD oil works by relaxing the body and then generating a low energy level so if you use it, you may find it easier for your heart rate to slow down a bit while also clearing your mind and enable you to have a restful and long sleep.

6. **CBD Improves Heart Health**

Recent findings from the Center for Disease Control and Prevention (CDC) show that heart disease is the **leading cause of death** around the world ahead of all other diseases with cancer coming in second. It is therefore very important to ensure that your heart is in good shape by ensuring that you make a healthy lifestyle and diet your priority while also supplementing that with some CBD oil.

It has shown to reduce artery blockage by widening clogged arteries while also protecting other blood vessels from getting damaged. It also reduces blood pressure, and can reduce stress induced cardiovascular response when one is anxious or stressed. Studies show that CBD, once ingested, has the ability to influence platelet aggregation and boost white blood cell function.

Another study published in the *British Journal of Clinical Pharmacology* in 2013 shows the function of CBD in preventing vascular damage that is brought about by inflammation, the induction of type 2 diabetes and a high glucose environment in animal models. In addition, it was discovered that CBD had the potential to lessen the vascular hyper-permeability, which is usually responsible for a leaky gut.

7. **CBD Lowers Prevalence Of Diabetes**

In a study conducted in 2006, scientists discovered that treating young non-obese mice with CBD significantly reduced their possibility of developing diabetes from an incidence percentage of 86% to 30%. Moreover, there was also a significant reduction in the plasma levels of inflammatory cytokines. When the scientists conducted a histological test of the pancreatic islets of the rodents they had treated with CBD, they discovered that insulitis had reduced significantly.

Another study that was published in the *American Journal of Medicine* brought to light the impact of cannabis use on insulin, glucose and insulin resistance in adults. This study comprised of 4,657 adult men and women from the (NHNES) National Health and Nutritional Examination Survey.

From that number, 1975 of them were identified as past cannabis users while 579 were current users.

Those who were current users were found to have 16% lower fasting insulin levels. Scientists also discovered a noteworthy connection between the use of cannabis and having a smaller waist circumference.

CBD has also been found to delay and inhibit the destruction of pancreatic cells that produce insulin. It also inhibits the production of inflammatory cytokines in people suffering from diabetes. All these findings strengthen the assumption that cannabidiol (which for your information is completely safe for human consumption regardless of potency or quantity) has all the attributes needed to be used as a therapeutic agent for treatment of type 1 diabetes when it has been discovered to develop from an early stage.

8. **CBD Promotes Healthy Weight**

Scientists have discovered that it is the over activation of the endocannabinoid system, especially through the activation of the CB1 receptors, that has been contributing to the increased abdominal obesity which is the accumulation of fatty tissues along the midsection. This, combined with the uptake of glucose into fatty cells and insulin resistance in the muscle tissues, can lead to metabolic dysfunction. And if not handled with the necessary attention it requires, one could find him/herself with more insulin resistance in their liver and muscles. With the victim struggling with an increased and uncontrollable appetite, this could lead to rapid and uncontainable body fat gain.

But there's a way to prevent and fight this massive weight gain. Professor Daniele Piomelli observes that the repeated use of CBD oil could eventually dull the CB1 receptors making them less sensitive. In due course, they eventually become inactive. It is therefore this weakening of these receptors that translates into a lower risk for obesity and even diabetes. This is due to the fact that the dormant receptor cannot be able to respond to the CBD cannabinoid molecules, which play an important role in allowing fat to accumulate in the body. This means that your high tolerance for CBD could be what is just keeping your blood sugar levels normal and body weight healthy.

There's also a recent study that reveals exactly how CBD impacts metabolism through a process known as *'fat browning',* which means the conversion of the White Adipose Tissue (usually white colored fatty tissue that stores energy) to the Brown Adipose Tissue (brown colored fatty tissue that burns it). The researchers tried to discover what would happen when preadipocytes (immature fat cells) were exposed to CBD. It was observed that CBD was:

- Found to increase the number of mitochondria and their functioning, therefore burning more calories
- Found to stimulate proteins and genes that are responsible for triggering oxidation to break down body fat
- Found to reduce the expression of proteins involved in lipogenesis (the production of new fatty cells)

9. **CBD Treats Skin Conditions**

When applied topically, CBD oil can be used to treat a variety of skin conditions. For instance, studies reveal that CBD has a slowing effect on proliferation and lipid synthesis of human sebaceous glands. It also has an anti-inflammatory effect on these glands. This means that cannabidiol can be used as a therapeutic agent for the cure of acne. CBD also reduces growth of (keratinocytes) skin cells thus preventing psoriasis.

10. CBD Prevents Neurodegenerative Diseases

Studies show that CBD is effective in preventing the toxic effects caused by ROS (radical oxygen species) and neurotransmitter glutamate in your brain thus preventing the death of brain cells. It also protects brain cells from beta-amyloid toxicity and for this reason, doctors believe that it could be used as a therapy for both Parkinson's and Alzheimer's diseases.

Since CBD possesses antioxidant and anti-inflammatory properties, scientists believe that it could be a promising therapeutic agent for the treatment of Amyotrophic Lateral Sclerosis (ALS).

11. CBD Cures Epilepsy

In one survey that involved parents of children suffering from epilepsy, about 84% of the parents reported that their children's seizures had reduced in frequency after using CBD. The children reported to have a better mood, increased alertness and better sleep although fatigue and drowsiness were some of the side effects they experienced.

The children were subjected to 3 months of treatment using a 98% oil-based and purified CBD extract. 39% of the children suffering from the condition were seen to have decreased their seizures by over 50%.

Now that you have a good understanding of the benefits that come with CBD, the next chapter will focus on how to find CBD oil to use it to derive the benefits.

Where to Find CBD Oil

If you are new to the CBD world, it can sometimes prove difficult to not only find where to purchase the oil, but also to find CBD rich oil. Some CBD oil sold by vendors is not effective in treating some of the ailments mentioned in the previous topic. This ineffectiveness is caused by the presence of impurities in the product. This is why you have to ensure that you get value for your money. To be honest, you will not find any retailer or manufacturer telling you that they sell low quality or mediocre oil. Instead, they'll be bragging about the benefits that you will get from their products. That said, there are a variety of ways you can find good quality cannabidiol oil:

1. **Brick and Mortar stores**

The good thing with buying CBD oil from these stores is that you are able to see or touch the product physically before buying it. This gives you the chance to inspect the packaging of the product and list of ingredients.

Buying over the counter offers you the chance to engage actively with the store vendor by asking questions about the various products to learn which one you might be interested in more. If you seek for a high quality and reputable vendor, it is very important that you inquire about 3rd party test results of the product. This is one way to be guaranteed that you will be purchasing a safe and high quality CBD oil because trustworthy manufacturers will want to invest in such tests to gain the trust of many clients.

Many retailers are free to sell what they consider to be the best form of CBD oil. The unscrupulous ones take advantage of the increasing demand for the product and sell those that contain a little or no cannabinoids at all. Beware that their dishonesty is fueled by the urge to make more money by sourcing the cheapest CBD oils in the black market and they do not have your best interests at heart.

2. **Dispensaries**

Just like the brick and mortar store, you can also visit the dispensary. The only difference is that dispensaries are more regulated by the state. For the dispensary to be operational, it must meet the following requirements:

- Must meet the health and safety standards as provided for by the law
- Must meet security requirements as well as
- Strict licensing guidelines

If you wish to purchase hemp-based CBD oil, you won't be required to show your card. However, to buy marijuana plant-based CBD oil, it is mandatory that you be certified by a doctor who is registered under the medical cannabis program of your state. Remember that the above will only apply to persons who only live in the states where medical marijuana laws have been passed.

When you visit your nearest dispensary, don't forget to ask for proof to show that the CBD products you are about to purchase have undergone lab tests and clinical trials. At the end of the day, it's you who will be consuming them anyway and you will need to ensure that they not only work but are safe for use.

3. **Online stores**

The third and last option is to purchase these products online and have them delivered at the comfort of your home. Most people prefer this method because it's a convenient, quick and secure way of having CBD oil delivered to your doorstep.

If you have no idea where to start, could begin by typing 'the best CBD oils for sale' on your favorite search engine. From there, a number of suggestions will be listed for you. Check each one of them. Although this may be a bit tedious, it's better than searching physically for retail stores.

Whenever you find an online vendor you like, chances are you'll be given a variety of their products to choose from. Here, you will have the luxury of choosing from the different alternatives in front of your screen. Another advantage is that you have the chance to compare product prices with other vendors and go for the cheaper option of the same or better quality.

One of the best advantages of purchasing online is that you can easily do some quick research about the products on sale by going through the product reviews, testimonials or social media platforms so as to determine the reputation of the manufacturer and product. This is one of the most reliable and effective ways to know how authentic the product you are about to buy is. By checking the product reviews, you will read some of the testimonials and even bad reviews of some of the clients who used that particular product. This will make your work easier because you will weigh the different options and make the best decision based on whichever product the users found to be most effective. If for instance you read many complaints about a certain product or vendor, then it's better if you just keep off.

In conclusion, ensure that you research more so that you may make an informed decision of buying the best product. Use your personal discretion at all times before purchasing a product online or over-the-counter. Moreover, most people always go for the cheaper products and end up getting substandard hemp oils. If you really want to enjoy the amazing benefits of a high quality cannabidiol extract, then you have no choice but to pay whatever price that is demanded of it. And most importantly, always check the labels for indication of the ingredients that make the product to make sure that it is indeed CBD oil from hemp. If it doesn't have any label, then it is illegal and potentially dangerous. Don't buy it.

Next, we will be discussing how to use the CBD oil that you've purchased.

How To Use CBD Oil

There are 4 main ways of introducing cannabinoids into your system. It's up to you to decide the best method for your convenience.

1. **Ingestion**

Swallowing is the easiest way of introducing a dose of CBD to a beginner or a child. There is no need to teach anyone how to swallow CBD oil or cannabidiol infused foods or drinks. When swallowed, the product passes through the entire digestive system and is metabolized in the liver. The active compound (cannabidiol) then seeps into the bloodstream just the same way all nutrients are delivered.

Most ingestible CBD oil comes in the form of capsules, tablets or pills. You will also find some CBD infused foods in the market such as pizza sauce, peanut butter, honey, chocolate bars, cookies and gummies. There are also a wide variety of CBD infused drinks such as juices. CBD is scentless and flavorless and some people love to add it as an ingredient as they cook their meals. CBD oil can also be added to beverages such as tea, coffee, liquid shots or smoothies. CBD edibles and drinks can take up to half an hour to reach the bloodstream.

2. **Sub-lingual Means**

The term sub-lingual means that you administer by placing the oil under the tongue. By placing CBD oil under your tongue, you allow the active compounds to get absorbed by the capillaries located in the mucous membrane and straight into the bloodstream. It has an immediate effect and is suitable for patients suffering from pain.

This method bypasses the digestive system. It therefore preserves the efficacy of the cannabinoid. CBD also avoids metabolism by the liver and therefore using only a little amount of the oil will still induce a stronger reaction from the compound. This is because the compound still remains intact even when entering into the bloodstream. The correct procedure is to read the label on the tincture bottle to know how many drops you will need to place under your tongue. Hold the CBD oil under your tongue for one or two minutes to enable the mucous membrane to exhaust all cannabinoids. Do not swallow.

3. **Inhalation/Vaping**

While this is the most efficient and fastest method of introducing CBD into the body, it is also the most complicated to master especially if you are teaching a non smoker. Once inhaled, the substance immediately enters the lungs and diffuses into the bloodstream therefore bypassing the liver and digestive system. This method is efficient because a large percentage of the original substance enters the bloodstream more as opposed to using other methods of administration. However, the compound also tends to also clear out of the bloodstream quicker.

4. **Topical Application**

You can also apply CBD oil enriched products on the skin. Such include lotions, balms, salves, gels oils, butters and trans-dermal patches. There are also CBD infused soaps, moisturizers and shampoos available.

When these products are used topically, the cannabinoids do not enter into the bloodstream with the only exception being trans-dermal patches. This means that they only work on the uppermost layer of the skin. If you rub some CBD lotion on your skin for example, the cannabinoid-carrying lipids in the lotion diffuse through the skin cell membranes and immediately, the CBD starts its healing, pain relieving and therapeutic mechanisms on the surrounding tissue and cell layers.

This is the best method to use if you need quick relief from muscle cramps, tension, fibromyalgia, arthritis or any other form of pain.

5. **Use Of Suppositories**

This is the least known method of administration but it's effective nevertheless. Suppositories are solid forms of CBD that are inserted into the rectum, urethra or vagina. They are a good way to deliver drugs in the body when other methods cannot be used.

Once inserted, the suppository dissolves to the rest of the body through the bloodstream. Studies show that receiving medication through the use of suppositories allows for a relatively constant environment for the substance to be delivered.

I know you may be wondering; are there any possible side effects? That's what we will be discussing next.

Possible Risks And Side Effects Involved

Like anything else in life, using CBD has its pros and cons. We've already discussed the pros so this chapter will focus on the cons.

1. **Drop In Blood Pressure**

When taken in large quantities, CBD can cause a slight drop in blood pressure and this usually happens a few minutes after administering the cannabidiol in your system. Therefore, if you may be taking medication for blood pressure, it is advisable that you consult with your physician before using CBD.

2. **Lightheadedness And Drowsiness**

This is a result of the drop in blood pressure. The lightheadedness is easily resolved by taking a cup of tea or coffee. If you feel drowsy after consuming CBD, do not drive or operate heavy machinery.

3. **Dry Mouth**

A 2006 study published by scientists from Argentina discovered the presence of type 1 and 2 cannabinoid receptors in the sub-mandibular glands that produce saliva. Whenever these receptors are activated by administering CBD in the body, the production of saliva is reduced. This leads to an unpleasant feeling of having a dry mouth, which is also known as 'cotton mouth'. This also triggers thirst.

4. **Increase In Tremor Frequency For Parkinson's Disease Patients**

If taken in large quantities, CBD can worsen muscle movement and tremors in Parkinson's disease sufferers. If this is witnessed, the amount of cannabinoid for the patient should be reduced to reduce the occurrence of this side effect. Overall, any patient suffering from this disease should consult his/her physician for advice before they start their CBD regimen with little doses.

Other possible side effects include sedation and the slowing of psycho-motor functions such as slowed movements and thoughts.

Conclusion

We have come to the end of the book. Thank you for reading and congratulations for reading until the end.

I truly hope you found the book educative and actionable. The most interesting thing about CBD is that it is 'nearly impossible' to overdose on it; the reason being that it has an unusually low level of toxicity. In fact, the use of cannabis, not only CBD – regardless of quantity or potency – cannot induce a fatal overdose. However, since there exists no FDA regulations for CBD oils, it is recommended that you seek advice from a medical professional to determine the best dosage for maximum benefits.

If you found the book valuable, can you recommend it to others? One way to do that is to post a review on Amazon.

Thank you and good luck!